Contents

WHO Study Group on Training in Diagnostic Ultrasound: Essentials, Principles and Standards

Philadelphia, USA, 22–26 March 1996

Members

Professor S. Bhargava, All India Institute of Medical Sciences, New Delhi, India

Professor C. Bruguera, Diagnostic Imaging Teaching Institute, Buenos Aires, Argentina

Dr G.G. Cerri, University of São Paulo, São Paulo, Brazil

Professor S.H. Eik-Nes, National Centre for Fetal Medicine, Trondheim University Hospital, Trondheim, Norway

Professor M.R. El-Meligy, Faculty of Medicine, Cairo University, Cairo, Egypt

Professor H.A. Gharbi, Department of Radiology, Children's Hospital, Tunis, Tunisia

Professor B.B. Goldberg, The Jefferson Ultrasound Research and Education Institute, Thomas Jefferson University Medical College and Hospital, Philadelphia, PA, USA (*Chairman*)

Professor H.T. Lutz, Department of Medicine, No.1 Medical Clinic, Bayreuth, Germany

Professor C.R.B. Merritt, Department of Radiology, Ochsner Clinic, New Orleans, LA, USA (*Rapporteur*)

Dr D.E. Robinson, Ultrasonic Laboratory, Division of Radiophysics, Commonwealth Scientific and Industrial Research Organisation, Chatswood, New South Wales, Australia

Mrs D. Szabunio, Ultrasound Department, Women's College Hospital, Toronto, Ontario, Canada

Dr M.W. Wachira, Department of Diagnostic Radiology, University of Nairobi, Nairobi, Kenya (*Vice-Chairman*)

Professor H. Watanabe, Kyoto Prefectural University of Medicine, Kyoto, Japan

Professor P.N.T. Wells, Department of Medical Physics and Bioengineering and University Department of Hospital Medicine, Bristol General Hospital, Bristol, England

Dr Xu Zhi-Zhang, Zhong Shan Hospital, Shanghai Medical University, Shanghai, China

Representatives of other organizations

International Federation for Medical and Biological Engineering

Dr P.A. Lewin, Department of Electrical and Computer Engineering and Biomedical Engineering and Science Institute, Drexel University, Philadelphia, PA, USA

International Society and Federation of Cardiology

Professor A.E. Belinsky, Buenos Aires, Argentina

International Society of Radiographers and Radiological Technologists

Ms C. Babiak, Michener Institute for Applied Health Sciences, Toronto, Ontario, Canada

International Society of Radiology

Dr P. Arger, Radiology Department, University Hospital of Pennsylvania, Philadelphia, PA, USA

Society of Diagnostic Medical Sonographers (USA)

Dr M. Berman, Roslyn Heights, NY, USA

World Federation of Sonographers

Dr R. Curry, Program Director, 1997 World Federation of Sonographers Meeting, Sickerville, NJ, USA

Ms K. Griffiths, President, World Federation of Sonographers, Dundas, Australia

World Federation for Ultrasound in Medicine and Biology

Professor A.E. Belinsky, Buenos Aires, Argentina

Secretariat

Dr S. Hancke, Head, Ultrasonic Laboratory, Gentofte Hospital, University of Copenhagen, Copenhagen, Denmark (*Temporary Adviser*)

Professor Emeritus P.E.S. Palmer, University of California, Davis, California, CA, USA (*Temporary Adviser*)

Dr V. Volodin, Medical Officer, Radiation Medicine, WHO, Geneva, Switzerland (*Secretary*)

Dr A. Wasunna, Director, Programme on Health Technology, WHO, Geneva, Switzerland

Professor M.C. Ziskin, Center for Biomedical Physics, Temple University School of Medicine, Philadelphia, PA, USA (*Temporary Adviser*)

1. Introduction

A WHO Study Group on Training in Diagnostic Ultrasound: Essentials, Principles and Standards met in Philadelphia, PA, USA, from 22 to 26 March 1996 to consider methods of improving the training and clinical performance of physicians and allied health professionals[1] who use ultrasound for diagnostic applications. The meeting was opened by Dr A. Wasunna, Director, Programme on Health Technology, WHO, Geneva, on behalf of the Director-General.

Diagnostic ultrasound is a rapidly developing imaging technology which is widely used in both industrialized and developing countries. Since its introduction in the 1960s, ultrasound has found widespread application in anatomical imaging, blood-flow measurement, and evaluation of physiology in almost all aspects of medicine (*1*). As ultrasound instruments have become smaller, less expensive, and easier to use, diagnostic ultrasound has become increasingly popular among a wide variety of physicians. Ultrasound imaging technique has replaced or complemented a large number of radiographic and nuclear medicine procedures and has opened new areas of diagnostic investigation (see Annex). For example, in many cardiovascular diseases diagnostic ultrasound has replaced invasive methods as the primary means of evaluation. In obstetrics, where radiography is no longer generally used, diagnostic ultrasound has provided an important means of assessing fetal viability and age, evaluating fetal development, and diagnosing fetal, uterine, and placental abnormalities. In some countries (e.g. Austria, Germany, Iceland and Norway), routine ultrasound examinations are offered through government programmes to all pregnant women during the second trimester. Ultrasound is considered as the primary imaging modality for the detection of most gynaecological, hepatic, biliary, pancreatic, splenic, and renal diseases and for examination of the scrotal contents, bladder, and prostate. In many developing countries, diagnostic ultrasound may find an important application as an epidemiological screening and diagnostic procedure for a number of parasitic diseases, such as amoebiasis, schistosomiasis, and echinococcosis.

Good medical practice requires ultrasonography practitioners to consider the risks and benefits of diagnostic examinations, and to take all proper measures to ensure maximum patient benefit with minimum risk. The use of diagnostic ultrasound should be encouraged where there is a likelihood of clinical benefit and discouraged in cases for

---

[1] Allied health professionals are recognized health professionals (e.g. sonographers, midwives, nurses) who are not physicians.

which no such benefit is expected (2). Ultrasonography has established an enviable safety record. There has not yet been any published report of harmful biological effects due to diagnostic ultrasound, on either patients or operators (3–6). As a result, there tends to be little regulation of diagnostic ultrasound equipment, which facilitates its acquisition. In fact, few countries currently regulate the use of diagnostic ultrasound. Moreover, diagnostic ultrasound equipment is less expensive than most other imaging equipment. The low cost and lack of regulation mean that diagnostic ultrasound equipment is often used by personnel without adequate training.

With the introduction of endovaginal, endorectal, transoesophageal, echocardiographic, intraoperative, pulsed and colour Doppler ultrasound and other specialized techniques, the difficulties of performing examinations and interpreting their results have significantly increased. The use of diagnostic ultrasound by individuals without proper training and experience adds to the likelihood of unnecessary examinations and misdiagnosis. The need for adequate education and training in ultrasonography exists in both industrialized and developing countries. Moreover, the challenge of providing adequate training in ultrasonography is made more difficult by the diversity of its utilization, since no single medical specialty has a monopoly on its use.

Diagnostic ultrasound is recognized as a safe, effective, and highly flexible imaging modality capable of providing clinically relevant information about most parts of the body in a rapid and cost-effective fashion. Obtaining maximum clinical benefit from diagnostic ultrasound, as well as ensuring the optimal utilization of health care resources, requires a combination of appropriate instrumentation and skills in both the performance and interpretation of examinations. The proper, safe, and effective use of diagnostic ultrasound is therefore highly dependent on the user, who has a major impact on the examination's overall benefit. In fact, the skill and training of the user are often more important than the equipment used. For this reason, standards for ultrasonography training are a prerequisite for the provision of diagnostic ultrasound services of high quality.

In view of ultrasonography's growth and the acquisition of equipment by those with minimal training, some patients may be harmed by misdiagnosis resulting from improper indications for use, poor examination technique, and errors in interpretation (7, 8).

1.1 Background to the Study Group's report

The purpose of this report is to define the essential training and skills necessary for the effective employment of diagnostic ultrasound in different health care settings. Preparation of the report has been guided by several WHO publications, including *Future use of new imaging technologies in developing countries: report of a WHO Scientific Group* (9), *Effective choices for diagnostic imaging in clinical practice: report of a WHO Scientific Group* (10) and *Manual of diagnostic ultrasound* (11), published in collaboration with the World Federation for Ultrasound in Medicine and Biology.

The WHO Scientific Group on Clinical Diagnostic Imaging commented on the wide variety of imaging techniques and the limited availability of some of these methods in certain parts of the world (10). Three levels of imaging equipment were described. Level I includes standard radiography equipment, as for the WHO Basic Radiological System (now called the World Health Imaging System for Radiography (WHIS-RAD))[1], general purpose diagnostic ultrasound equipment, and equipment for conventional linear tomography and for fluoroscopy with image intensification. Level II includes level I equipment and techniques plus sophisticated radiography, sophisticated ultrasonography (including Doppler), mammography, angiography, digital subtraction angiography (DSA), macro-radiography, computerized tomography (CT), radionuclide scintigraphy (including single-photon emission computerized tomography (SPECT)), and thermography. Level III includes all level I and II equipment and techniques, as well as magnetic resonance imaging (MRI), positron emission tomography (PET), and advanced radionuclide scanning with labelling by means of monoclonal antibodies (immunoscintigraphy). Level I resources are typical of many parts of the world; level II and III resources are usually found only in affluent regions. Ultrasonography is recognized as important for good patient care at each of these levels, whether it be general ultrasonography at level I centres or advanced ultrasonography, including Doppler techniques, at level II and III centres.

As stated by the WHO Scientific Group on Clinical Diagnostic Imaging, "more important than the equipment is the availability of skills. An error in diagnosis because of inadequate education and experience is as dangerous as being without the equipment, and the success of any interventional procedure (e.g. angiography) is very dependent on the skill and experience of the responsible physician." The Scientific Group further noted that "in particular, the effective use of an ultrasound scanner, although less expensive than other imaging equipment, is very dependent on the physician" (10).

---

[1] Details for WHIS-RAD can be found in *Technical specifications for the World Health Imaging System for Radiography — the WHIS-RAD*. Geneva, World Health Organization, 1995 (unpublished document WHO/RAD/TS/95.1; available on request from Programme on Health Technology, World Health Organization, 1211 Geneva 27, Switzerland).

According to the WHO Scientific Group on the Future Use of New Imaging Technologies in Developing Countries, a general physician should perform a minimum of 200 obstetric and abdominal examinations with a general purpose ultrasound scanner before he or she can be considered able to interpret scans with any reliability. However, for a physician to become a competent sonologist,[1] the Group recommended at least 6 months' full-time training in a recognized centre, with additional experience being advisable (9). The present Study Group has reviewed these and other recommendations in the light of recent progress in ultrasonography.

The Scientific Group on the Future Use of New Imaging Technologies in Developing Countries also noted that "the difficulties in making an accurate diagnosis from ultrasound images are such that the purchase of ultrasound equipment without making provision for the training of an operator is contrary to good health care practice and is unlikely to be cost-effective". This same Scientific Group recommended that "wherever possible, ultrasound examinations should be carried out by trained physicians", and went on to add that, if non-physicians are to perform examinations, they need to have at least a year's full-time training and should always work under the supervision of an experienced sonologist. These recommendations were endorsed by the authors of the *Manual of diagnostic ultrasound* and reflect the opinion of this Study Group as well.

The need for training in the use of diagnostic ultrasound for community-based surveys to evaluate morbidity due to schistosomiasis was stressed in the recommendations of a WHO Expert Committee's report *The control of schistosomiasis* (12). The importance of ultrasound in the surveillance and management of problems related to echinococcosis has also been noted (13).

Properly developed programmes for training physicians and allied health professionals in ultrasonography exist in only a few industrialized countries (14). There are no detailed international recommendations or guidance for training those who are using or wish to use this imaging technique. It was partly for these reasons that WHO prepared the *Manual of diagnostic ultrasound*, which provides guidance on the ultrasound diagnosis of a wide variety of common conditions at the primary and first-referral levels of health care. It is intended for use by physicians, sonographers,[2] nurses, and midwives with basic training in ultrasonography, working with a general purpose ultra-

---

[1] A sonologist is a physician qualified to perform and interpret ultrasound examinations.
[2] A sonographer is a technician qualified to perform assigned ultrasound examinations and procedures (see p. 21).

sound scanner, but without ready access to expert advice. However, the manual is not intended to be a textbook on diagnostic ultrasound and should not be considered to replace the need for proper training.

1.2 Structure of the report

Section 2 of this report reviews the present situation in ultrasonography and trends in the utilization of diagnostic ultrasound in clinical practice. It also examines worldwide practice with respect to ultrasonography training for physicians, sonographers and other categories of medical professionals (e.g. midwives, nurses, assistant physicians). Section 3 presents outlines of recommended training curricula for physicians in general, advanced, and specialized ultrasonography and discusses various other factors that must be taken into account in organizing the training process. Section 4 describes the recommended training for allied health professionals specializing in ultrasonography. Section 5 presents the basic science and instrumentation aspects of the curricula described in sections 3 and 4. The various sections of the report, and in particular section 6, discuss the level of competence that should be reached by those trained in the use of diagnostic ultrasound, as well as the recommended standards for training programmes and the training process, including the recommended requirements for instructors and training centres. Section 7 summarizes the recommendations of the Study Group.

It is recognized that some of the principles and approaches used in training in the use of diagnostic ultrasound still require further clarification, and that in some countries it may be difficult to apply certain recommendations in full. The Study Group regards the curricula presented here as the minimum that should be required everywhere; however, even partial implementation of the recommendations made here would represent progress in training and improved clinical utilization of this useful technology.

2. The world situation with respect to ultrasonography

2.1 Assessment of current practice

2.1.1 Performance and interpretation

The earliest clinical uses of diagnostic ultrasound were for evaluation of the uterus during pregnancy, and of the breast, abdomen, heart, and pelvic organs, and were pioneered by physicians and researchers from a number of specialties (1). The introduction of

Doppler ultrasound for the evaluation of blood flow in the 1970s made possible additional clinical applications. With the development of specialized instruments for endovaginal, endorectal, endo-oesophageal, and intravascular (endoluminal) scanning, ultrasound has been adopted by a broad range of medical specialties and is now an essential method of diagnosis and guidance for intervention or therapy in many fields. The Annex summarizes by specialty the common applications of diagnostic ultrasound.

The versatility of ultrasonography in aiding the diagnosis of a broad range of diseases, coupled with the widespread availability of relatively low-cost general purpose scanners with good performance, has encouraged the use of diagnostic ultrasound throughout general medicine and paediatric practice and other specialties. The level of knowledge and training on the part of practitioners is accordingly highly diverse (*14–19*).

Although ultrasound examinations are generally performed and interpreted by physicians, in some parts of the world allied health professionals, including sonographers and midwives, are responsible for the performance of ultrasound imaging. However, the interpretation of abnormal ultrasound images and diagnostic decision-making are the responsibility of physicians in all countries.

2.1.2 *Delivery of services*

Previous WHO publications have included basic ultrasonography with diagnostic radiography as essential elements of basic diagnostic imaging services. The relatively compact size of general purpose ultrasound units, their uncomplicated power requirements, and their portability permit the delivery of diagnostic ultrasound services in a variety of settings where other imaging modalities cannot be employed. Training requirements for practitioners of ultrasonography must therefore provide not only for specialized users in well equipped medical centres, but also for practitioners in remote environments.

In level I settings, ultrasound services are likely to be provided in a clinic or hospital by a general physician or in some cases by a midwife.

In level II and III settings, ultrasonography is likely to be practised in a radiology department or by a clinical ultrasound specialist, often using equipment with special features such as Doppler and colour Doppler, or endoluminal transducers. In some countries sonographers are responsible for the performance of such examinations.

Worldwide, there is great variation in both the sophistication of ultrasound equipment and the qualifications of those providing diagnostic ultrasound services. In addition to its use in general medicine, ultrasonography is practised by a variety of specialists, including radiologists and sonologists, and is consequently used for a wide range of examinations. An indication of training needs according to the availability of diagnostic imaging equipment is given in Table 1.

2.1.3 *Equipment and techniques*

WHO has published specifications for a general purpose ultrasound scanner (*9, 11*). This is a general purpose imaging unit without Doppler or flow-imaging capability, and is recommended as suitable for a medical centre with standard X-ray equipment, such as the WHO Basic Radiological System (now called the World Health Imaging System for Radiography; see footnote, p. 3). Such a combination is typical of most parts of the world. More sophisticated diagnostic ultrasound, including pulsed spectral Doppler and colour Doppler and specialized probes for endovaginal, endorectal, endo-oesophageal, intraoperative, laparascopic, and endoluminal applications, is available in more affluent areas of the world, usually in the hands of specialists.

2.1.4 *Recognized indications for ultrasonography*

Clinical conditions for which diagnostic ultrasound is generally recognized as the imaging procedure of choice have been described elsewhere (*10*). In addition, diagnostic ultrasound is recognized as a primary or secondary imaging procedure in a broad range of clinical situations.

Table 1

Ultrasound training needs according to equipment availability

Level of equipment	Level of training required	Professional category	
		General	Specialized
I	Sufficient to perform common examinations safely and accurately	Family physician, trauma physician, sonographer	Midwife, paediatrician
II	Sufficient to accept and manage referrals	Radiologist, sonologist	Obstetrician/gynaecologist, cardiologist, other specialists (see Annex)
III	Advanced, for teaching and research	Radiologist (organ-oriented sub-specialties), sonologist	Advanced specialists (perinatologists and sub-specialized internists and surgeons)

2.2 Trends in ultrasonography

Important trends in the use of diagnostic ultrasound include a growing recognition of its cost-effectiveness and importance in clinical problem-solving. This has resulted in its increased use for both diagnostic and interventional procedures. At the same time, the performance, reliability, and flexibility of ultrasound scanners have increased, resulting in lower costs per unit of performance. Thus, both the complexity of ultrasound equipment and the variety of its uses are increasing throughout the world.

However, because of the variability in training, the quality of diagnosis is improving in some areas but declining in others. An important factor is that the rate of change in technology and the pattern of utilization is not being met by the increased production of a sufficient number of trained users in many parts of the world. The lack of uniform and generally accepted standards for training compounds the problem.

2.3 Current ultrasonography training

Worldwide, it is likely that much of the ultrasonography currently performed is carried out by individuals with in fact little or no formal training. Further, the need for basic training is greater in developing than in developed countries. Wherever users have little or no formal training in ultrasound principles, clinical examination techniques, or diagnosis, training should be a priority, as a significant benefit in health care will result from improved skills in the performance and interpretation of ultrasound examinations.

In some developed countries, ultrasonography is included as a part of formal training in several medical specialties, including radiology, cardiology, obstetrics, and surgery (*20, 21*). However, uniform standards for training physicians do not generally exist (*22*). Many ultrasonography practitioners do not have adequate experience, and an even greater number would benefit from additional training. However, educational opportunities are often limited, and a standard curriculum to ensure the mastery of minimum essential skills has not been defined. In developed countries the greatest need is for training to maintain and increase levels of competence, whereas in developing countries both entry-level training and continuing education are primary needs (*15, 16, 18, 19, 23*).

2.4 Variations in training and practice

In most countries, trainees in diagnostic imaging (i.e. radiology) are required to learn and understand the use of diagnostic ultrasound in all clinical situations. In most radiology training programmes in the United States, at least 3 months but usually more are devoted entirely to ultrasonography. After completion of specialized training, many radiologists in the United States continue for an additional year of advanced ultrasonography training. In other countries, ultrasonography training requirements may be more (e.g. Israel), or less demanding (e.g. Turkey). In non-imaging specialties, training requirements also vary. Scandinavian countries require courses of 30 hours of ultrasonography training for obstetrics, 20 hours for cardiology, and 24 hours for gastroenterology.

There is similar variation among those who practise ultrasonography. For instance, in Germany, ultrasound scanning is performed exclusively by physicians; at present, no allied health professionals may use diagnostic ultrasound either alone or under supervision. Many ultrasound examinations in Germany are carried out in private (non-hospital) practice (more than 18 million in 1994). Ultrasonography training for German physicians forms part of their internship, and consists of theory and practice components, often directed towards the specialty they will practise. Post-training evaluation is rare, but the organization of training programmes is well established. The training guidelines and quality control measures aimed to ensure the skills of those practising ultrasonography have been created by the German health insurance system, not by a medical or academic body (24).

In Japan, the Japanese Society of Ultrasound Medicine has formed a group of teacher/physicians responsible for the training of doctors and other health professionals applying for accreditation in ultrasonography. This accreditation has not yet been accorded an official status.

In Australia and New Zealand, the Australasian Society for Ultrasound in Medicine (ASUM) in 1970 formally recognized the need for comprehensive education to ensure high quality practice in ultrasonography (19). Diplomas were established for sonologists (1976) and sonographers (1979); these diplomas have effectively become prerequisites for those providing training in ultrasonography. Nevertheless, as in Japan, there is still no legal accreditation requirement for those practising ultrasonography. A system of self-regulation operates within medical colleges (associations), whose members constitute the majority of ultrasonography practitioners. Non-members are not, however, subject to the same requirements.

In the United Kingdom, ultrasonography is a component of training in radiology, which is restricted to those having at least 2 years of training in general medicine. In addition, radiologists are trained only at centres accredited by the Royal College of Radiologists, which is also responsible for continuing medical education in the field. Joint programmes with other Royal Colleges, such as the Royal College of Obstetricians and Gynaecologists, are also being organized to provide advanced training in ultrasonography. Participants in these training programmes must attend 100 ultrasound sessions comprising a total of 300 hours of instruction. Training in cardiac ultrasonography is provided by the British Society of Echocardiography, affiliated to the British Cardiac Society, which has established levels of required training and education. The requirements include attendance at not less than 100 examinations per year after completion of training.

In Latin America, several different approaches to training exist. In some countries, ultrasonography is taught during specialized medical training, and consequently reaches only newly qualified physicians. Such training includes a required course in theory and 1000 practical examinations under supervision. For advanced specialization in ultrasound, short (1–3 months) and long (6–12 months) courses exist, as well as 1-week refresher courses.

In China, training schemes for both general and advanced ultrasonography exist, and can be attended at various stages of the medical career (e.g. post-graduate, fellowship). Continuing education programmes are currently being established. Similar training patterns exist in only a few other developing countries (e.g. India).

In the rest of the developing world, however, the situation is quite different. Diagnostic ultrasound services are often not available at all, or only at an inadequate level. They may be general ultrasonography services, for specific applications (e.g. obstetrics), or oriented towards problems such as hepatic parasites, urinary disease, or gastrointestinal infections and infestations. The equipment is often old or inadequate, because of a lack of funds. Consequently, it can be technically out of date, or suffer from poor maintenance and unavailability of spare parts. There are very few formal training programmes in ultrasonography, with the exception of some centres where radiologists are trained at university hospitals. Radiological societies may organize short refresher courses, but in much of the developing world adequate ultrasonography training or services are lacking. The accreditation of users and the control of quality are also rare.

2.5 Sonographers

Relatively few countries (e.g. Australia, Canada, Japan, New Zealand, the United Kingdom, and the United States) have well recognized and established guidelines and requirements for training sonographers (*25–28*). In most other countries, ultrasonography is performed exclusively by physicians, with the occasional exception of midwives (e.g. in Scandinavian countries). Where established training programmes for sonographers and midwives exist, they are comprehensive and require very high standards of knowledge and practice (see for example *18, 19, 25–27*).

2.6 Trends in ultrasonography training

Awareness of the need for ultrasonography training is increasing, and there are growing opportunities for the formal training and accreditation of both physicians and allied health professionals, particularly in developed countries.

New technologies such as electronic media, global telecommunications, and the Internet make possible novel approaches to training. In developed countries, requirements for continuing medical education to maintain and increase levels of competence, particularly in specialized areas, are increasing. In some countries, changes in health care practices and medical regulations are stimulating the institution of formal accreditation programmes for physicians and allied health professionals, as well as the accreditation of diagnostic services, including diagnostic ultrasound services.

3. Ultrasonography curricula for medical students and physicians

3.1 Curriculum for medical students

In view of the importance of ultrasonography as a primary diagnostic imaging method, all medical students should receive an introduction to its principles and uses, as well as to the relevant anatomy. Although this training need not be extensive, it should include at least:

- the basic principles of ultrasound imaging and its differences from radiographic and other methods, including the use of mechanical (acoustic) energy rather than ionizing electromagnetic energy;
- the anatomy of the axial, longitudinal, and coronal planes examined in ultrasound scanning, with special emphasis on the sectional anatomy of the abdomen and pelvis;
- a review of the major clinical indications and applications of ultrasound in diagnosis and intervention and the relationship of ultrasound to other imaging modalities, including cyst/solid differentiation and real-time features.

Evaluation of knowledge of ultrasonography, both theoretical and practical, should be included in the evaluation of medical students.

3.2 Curriculum for general (level I) ultrasonography for physicians

In level I settings, diagnostic ultrasound examinations are likely to be performed by a general physician using a general purpose ultrasound scanner. These physicians will be expected to perform safely and accurately a variety of examinations of all parts of the body. The curriculum for training physicians must therefore include instruction in the performance and interpretation of diagnostic ultrasound examinations, and related areas of physics and instrumentation.

3.2.1 *General features of the curriculum*

Basic physical principles
The physical principles relating to ultrasound and its interaction with tissues that should be covered in the general curriculum are outlined in section 5.3. These include basic terminology, the physics of waves and their interaction with different tissues of the body, including amplitude, intensity, attenuation, perpendicular and oblique incidence, and scattering, the range equation, transducer construction and its effect on ultrasound waves, methods of focusing and resolution, useful frequency ranges, artefacts, biological effects, and safety.

Principles of scanning
The trainee should become familiar with:

- orientation of the image for standard display formats (head/foot and right/left orientation) and image annotation;
- image background (light echoes on a dark background versus dark echoes on a light background);
- scanning planes (sagittal, parasagittal, axial, coronal, and oblique) and image annotation for the scanning planes;
- proper adjustment of equipment controls (system gain, time gain compensation (TGC), depth of field of view, and focal zone placement);
- protocols for routine examinations, including standard transducers, the area to be imaged, and any required measurements and documentation;
- frequency, resolution, and their relationship;
- the recognition and identification of common artefacts and strategies to reduce or eliminate them, as well as recognition of artefacts that can enhance diagnostic accuracy;
- permanent image documentation.

Anatomy
The trainee should master:

- basic anatomy as visualized with ultrasound, with an emphasis on the anatomy of abdominal, pelvic, and fetal structures, soft tissue anatomy, and major vascular structures;
- sectional anatomy, including the relationships of major structures in the sagittal, axial, and coronal planes;
- normal anatomical size and position;
- common anatomical variations;
- normal fetal anatomy.

Pathology
The training should cover congenital, inflammatory, degenerative, metabolic, and neoplastic pathology and pathophysiology and common traumatic conditions affecting the major organs, soft tissues, and vascular structures.

The general indications for and limitations of ultrasonography should be taught.

The basic diagnostic criteria for the interpretation of scans should be covered, including tissue characteristics, normal and abnormal organ tissue patterns, and the differentiation of cystic and solid masses.

Standard methods for the reporting and documentation of results should be covered.

3.2.2 *Specific content*

The following presents the specific content that should be covered in the general ultrasonography curriculum, according to principal anatomical region (abdomen, chest, etc.). Physicians successfully completing the course should be able — safely, accurately, and consistently — to recognize the ultrasonographic appearance of the named structures or features, diagnose the conditions specified below, and perform the evaluations and measurements referred to. Variations in ultrasonographic appearance related to age and sex should be included in the course content as appropriate.

Abdomen

- Liver:
  - size and shape;
  - parenchyma;
  - intrahepatic vessels;

— focal lesions, including cysts, abscesses, tumours, trauma, and parasites;
— perihepatic fluid collections;
— normal and abnormal echogenicity (including both focal and diffuse disease).

- Gallbladder and biliary tract:
  — gallbladder size, wall, and contents, including calculi and *Ascaris*;
  — biliary tract dilatation and evaluation of the jaundiced patient;
  — normal bile duct measurements and physiological variations.
- Pancreas:
  — normal and abnormal echogenicity;
  — diffuse pancreatic disease;
  — focal lesions, including cysts, abscesses, tumours, and calcifications.
- Spleen:
  — size and shape;
  — focal lesions;
  — trauma.
- Kidneys and adrenals:
  — size, shape, and location;
  — diffuse parenchymal disease;
  — focal lesions, including cysts, tumours, and calculi;
  — obstructive uropathy and perirenal fluid collections.
- Ureters and bladder:
  — obstruction;
  — parasites;
  — tumours;
  — infections;
  — diverticula;
  — calculi.
- Peritoneal cavity and gastrointestinal tract:
  — intraperitoneal fluid collections;
  — bowel masses;
  — obstruction;
  — intussusception;
  — pyloric stenosis.
- Retroperitoneal space:
  — masses;
  — adenopathy;
  — fluid collections.
- Major abdominal vessels:
  — normal measurements;

— aortic aneurysm;
— inferior vena cava thrombus.

Chest

- Diaphragm.
- Subdiaphragmatic and supradiaphragmatic fluid collections.
- Pleural effusions, masses, and thickening.
- Peripheral lung masses.
- Gross mediastinal adenopathy.
- Thymus.

Female pelvis

- Normal physiological changes in the uterus and ovaries.
- Diseases of the urinary bladder, uterus, ovaries, fallopian tubes, and related blood vessels, muscles, and ligaments.
- Cystic, solid, and complex masses as well as inflammatory conditions, haematocolpos, endometriosis, and related gynaecological complications.

Note: Endovaginal techniques should not be included in this course.

Obstetrics

- Normal first trimester:
  — embryonic and early fetal anatomy;
  — yolk sac;
  — amniotic and chorionic cavities;
  — biometry including crown–rump length, amniotic sac diameter, and yolk sac size;
  — multiple pregnancy;
  — cardiac activity and confirmation of viability.
- Abnormal first trimester:
  — ectopic pregnancy;
  — complete and incomplete abortion;
  — vaginal bleeding;
  — fetal death;
  — hydatidiform mole;
  — major recognizable fetal malformations and developmental abnormalities (e.g. anencephaly);
  — pelvic mass.
- Second and third trimester:
  — development of fetal anatomy;
  — placenta (location and size) and umbilical cord (including two-vessel cord and location of cord insertion);
  — biometry of the cranium, abdomen, and femur;

   — assessment of fetal age;
   — amniotic fluid volume (normal volume and causes and criteria for diagnosis of oligohydramnios and polyhydramnios);
   — intrauterine growth retardation;
   — gross fetal abnormalities, including anencephaly, hydrocephalus, neural tube defects, abdominal wall defects, renal anomalies, and limb shortening.

Other applications

- Thyroid gland.
- Scrotal contents.
- Breast (both the muscles and the subcutaneous tissues for masses, abscesses, and abnormal fluid collections).
- Osteomyelitis, fractures, and callus.

Neonatal scanning

- Hydrocephalus.
- Pyloric stenosis.
- Abdominal masses.
- Hydronephrosis.
- Bladder abnormalities.
- Adrenal masses.
- Haemorrhage.
- Congenital hip dislocation.

3.2.3 Duration of training and required number of studies

The training programme should include lectures and practical demonstrations running over a period of 3–6 months, and the trainee should participate in 300–500 ultrasound examinations during this period. The practical demonstrations should include examinations appropriate for the disease profile of the country or region where the training is conducted. In most countries, an appropriate distribution of examinations would be:

- abdominal examinations (50%);
- obstetric examinations (20%);
- gynaecological examinations (20%);
- examinations of other parts (10%).

3.2.4 Evaluation

At the end of the course the trainee should be assessed by a recognized competent authority (see section 6) in both theoretical and practical aspects of ultrasonography and, if successful, accredited.

3.2.5 *Continuing medical education*

Continuing medical education that keeps the practitioner abreast of advances in technology and clinical practice is highly recommended.

3.3 Curriculum for advanced (level II and III) ultrasonography for physicians

3.3.1 *Purpose*

The purpose of the advanced ultrasonography curriculum for physicians is to ensure a level of training sufficient to perform high quality ultrasound examinations, using, when necessary, the more sophisticated ultrasound equipment available at levels II and III (which may correspond to the secondary and tertiary levels of health care in some countries). The physician successfully completing the curriculum should be able to perform all routine ultrasound examinations and also receive referred patients.

3.3.2 *Prerequisites*

The trainee should be a physician engaged in clinical practice as a generalist or specialist.

3.3.3 *Areas covered*

The curriculum should develop the necessary skills in physics, abdominal imaging, obstetrics, gynaecological examinations, and the scanning of other parts. Doppler, endovaginal, endorectal, and interventional procedures should be included.

3.3.4 *Content and duration*

The following material should be mastered:

- advanced-level physics of ultrasound imaging: terminology, artefacts, the biological effects of ultrasound (safety), and advanced-level Doppler theory (see section 5.4);
- instrumentation and equipment operation, set-up, and quality assurance (including issues related to endoluminal scanning);
- advanced ultrasound examination techniques and procedures, including control of infection;
- detailed cross-sectional anatomy;
- indications for and limitations of ultrasonography;
- criteria for diagnostic interpretation (including difficult and complicated cases);
- ultrasonically guided aspiration and biopsy;
- methods of reporting and documentation.

The curriculum should include both theoretical and practical aspects of advanced-level ultrasonography. The period of training should be at least 3 years (full time), if the trainee has not completed prior postgraduate medical training (specialization). If the trainee has already successfully completed a training programme in radiology, 3–9 months of additional training in ultrasonography are recommended. If the trainee has successfully completed postgraduate medical training in a field other than radiology, 1–2 years of additional training are advised.

For trainees who have not already qualified as radiologists, the theoretical component of the programme should include advanced-level physics and instrumentation. The statistics, computer science, pathology, pathophysiology, paediatrics, cross-sectional anatomy, surgery, and internal medicine that would normally be covered in a radiology training programme should also be included.

3.3.5 *Practical training*

During practical training, the trainee should perform a broad range of examinations under the supervision of experienced sonologists. These examinations should include those appropriate for the disease profile of the country or region in which the training is conducted. In most countries, an appropriate distribution would be:

- abdominal examinations (30%);
- obstetric examinations (20%);
- gynaecological examinations (10%);
- paediatric examinations (10%);
- examinations of peripheral vascular structures (15%);
- echocardiographic examinations (5%);
- examinations of other parts (10%).

Doppler, endovaginal, endorectal, and endo-oesophageal examinations and interventional ultrasound procedures should be included as appropriate.

3.3.6 *Evaluation*

At the end of the course, the trainee should be required to pass written, oral, and practical examinations, covering both theoretical and practical aspects. Upon successful completion of the examinations, the trainee should be granted the appropriate accreditation.

3.3.7 *Continuing medical education*

Continuing medical education that keeps the practitioner abreast of the latest advances in technology is highly recommended.

 Ultrasound in various specialties

Diagnostic ultrasound is used in many medical specialties, and specific training is recommended for clinical-imaging specialists in certain areas. In many cases, these specialists will have access to equipment with more capability than the general purpose ultrasound scanner, with features such as pulsed and colour Doppler and transducers with interventional capability. For the use of diagnostic ultrasound in one of the fields named below, training should include:

- the basic sciences and instrumentation curriculum for advanced ultrasonography (see section 5.4);
- detailed knowledge of the anatomy, pathology, and physiology related to the specialty;
- instruction in the ultrasound techniques and equipment relevant to the specialty.

In addition, training should:

- ensure participation in a sufficient number of specialized ultrasound examinations to attain and maintain proficiency;
- emphasize the need for continuing medical education;
- encourage formal documentation of competence in performance and interpretation of examinations;
- be carried out at an authorized centre for an adequate period of time (to be defined according to the requirements of various specialties).

The following sections present the additional material that is required for the use of diagnostic ultrasound in the named specialties.

Obstetrics and gynaecology

- Detailed embryonic and fetal anatomy.
- Diagnosis and management of fetal, uterine, and placental anomalies.
- Where appropriate, instruction in fetal blood sampling, fetal blood transfusion, chorionic villus sampling, and other invasive procedures performed under ultrasonic guidance.
- Detailed examination of the organs of the female pelvis, including the uterus, ovaries, and pelvic vessels; endovaginal examinations and interventional procedures.
- Detailed breast examinations, including ultrasonically guided biopsy.

Cardiology

- Detailed normal and abnormal cardiac anatomy.
- Detailed cardiac physiology, pathophysiology, and pathology.

- Evaluation of cardiac chamber size and dynamics, diagnosis of valvular and pericardial disease, measurement of blood pressure gradients, determination of blood flow volumes, detection and assessment of valvular regurgitation, demonstration and quantification of intracardiac shunts, and detection of intracavitary masses.
- Detailed instruction in M-mode, two-dimensional, and Doppler imaging techniques.
- Where appropriate, the techniques and interpretation of stress echocardiography, transoesophageal scanning, and the use of contrast media.

Note: Ultrasonography training for paediatric echocardiography should cover the same material.

Urology

- Detailed instruction in the anatomy, physiology, and pathology of the adrenals, kidneys, urinary bladder, prostate and seminal vesicles, urethra, penis, and scrotal contents.
- Instruction in techniques of intracavitary scanning of the bladder, transrectal scanning and interventional procedures using ultrasonic guidance; endovaginal scanning.
- Where appropriate, colour Doppler imaging and the use of contrast agents should be covered.

Gastroenterology

- Endoscopic ultrasound of the mediastinal gastrointestinal tract, liver, biliary tree, and pancreas.
- Endoscopic examination of the bile and pancreatic ducts.
- Where appropriate, interventional ultrasound techniques and Doppler imaging with contrast agents.

Internal medicine

- The use of Doppler ultrasound and appropriate interventional procedures.
- Echocardiography and training in the diagnosis of diseases of the visceral and peripheral arteries and veins may be included as appropriate.

Surgery

- Interventional, laparoscopic, and intraoperative ultrasound.
- Musculoskeletal examinations, as appropriate.

4. Ultrasonography training for sonographers and other allied health professionals

4.1 Introduction

The practice of ultrasonography varies throughout the world. In some countries, scanning can be carried out by trained allied health professionals under the supervision of physicians, but in others only physicians perform examinations. Allied health professionals include nurses and nurse/midwives, radiographers, nuclear medicine technologists, assistant physicians, and cardiac and vascular technologists (*15, 16, 28*). Where ultrasound is used extensively, as in obstetrics, allied health professionals have proved to be very effective in delivering diagnostic ultrasound services (*29, 30*). In specialized clinical areas such as echocardiography and vascular or ophthalmic ultrasound, such personnel can be extremely helpful for both patient and doctor. However, since the effectiveness of ultrasonography is highly dependent on the skill of the operator, this assistance requires extensive training.

4.2 A definition of a sonographer

In some countries the profession of "sonographer" has been recognized (*26, 27, 31*). The definition in one such country is as follows:

> Sonographers are highly skilled professionals qualified by technological education to provide patient services using diagnostic ultrasound under the supervision of a doctor of medicine. Sonographers or allied health personnel provide this service in a variety of medical settings, where the physician is responsible for the use and interpretation of ultrasound procedures. Sonographers and other allied health personnel assist physicians in gathering sonographic data necessary to reach diagnostic decisions (*25*).

The same definition also states that "the profession of diagnostic medical sonography includes general sonography, cardiac sonography, and various subspecialties. The profession requires judgment and the ability to provide appropriate health care services". This definition is given as an example; other countries may wish to establish their own definition of and criteria for professional sonographers.

4.3 Limitation of practice

Although sonographers are well trained and highly skilled, responsibility for the interpretation and reporting of the results of ultrasound examinations (apart from confirmation of normality), as well as the legal responsibility for all aspects of patient care, necessarily rests with the supervising physician. In most countries, endoluminal and endocavitary ultrasound examinations are performed by physicians only, but in some countries these studies can be carried out by sonographers. In all countries, however, interventional ultrasound, including biopsy, drainage, therapy, and amniocentesis, is performed exclusively by physicians.

4.4 Curriculum for general (level I) ultrasonography for sonographers and other allied health professionals

4.4.1 *Purpose*

The purpose of the general ultrasonography curriculum for sonographers and other allied health professionals is to ensure that users of diagnostic ultrasound have sufficient training to provide high quality health care. Training in the curriculum should result in an appropriate level of technical and clinical knowledge.

4.4.2 *Prerequisites*

Candidates for training should have completed 2–3 years of health care training, including courses in anatomy, physiology, and pathology.

If the candidate enters training directly from the secondary school level, it will then be necessary to provide supplementary education prior to ultrasonography training. The supplementary education should include sufficient instruction in anatomy, physiology, pathology, medical ethics, and physics for the practice of ultrasonography.

4.4.3 *General and specialized training*

Training may, as appropriate, be either general or specialized. In some clinical areas, specialized training may have to follow general training, but in others specialized training may be initiated directly. The training programme should consequently be structured appropriately.

The ultrasonography curriculum should provide for adequate time for the acquisition of clinical skills, and should require a specified number and range of ultrasound examinations. Protocols for the performance of ultrasound examinations are an important means of maintaining quality; because disease patterns vary, diagnostic medical departments or preferably national governments should establish examination protocols that sonographers and other allied health personnel should follow.

4.4.4 *Curriculum*

The curriculum for training sonographers and other allied health professionals is the same as the general curriculum for physicians, with the exceptions that the diagnostic conclusions and the reporting and documentation of the results of examinations are the responsibility of physicians.

4.4.5 *Duration of training and required number of studies*

The number of examinations necessary to ensure competence can vary for different applications of diagnostic ultrasound. Various physicians' and allied health professionals' organizations have established minimum numbers of ultrasound examinations in a number of specific areas. There is, however, no generally accepted number of examinations required to achieve proficiency. The following may serve as a guide:

* abdominal examinations (250);
* examinations of the neck (25);
* examinations of scrotal contents (25);
* pelvic examinations (50);
* first trimester pregnancy examinations (50);
* second and third trimester examinations (200);
* neonatal examinations (50).

The actual number required in a given curriculum may depend on the geographical area, the educational setting, and the disease profile of the population.

If endovaginal examinations are performed, the use of aseptic technique is very important, and additional training for this type of procedure should be offered.

4.4.6 *Clinical and ancillary information*

In addition to the topics of the general ultrasonography curriculum, the following should be covered:

* *Medical history.* How to obtain and describe a medical history, including laboratory or other test values related to the examination.
* *Patient preparation and care.* Patients should be informed about how to prepare for an examination by ultrasound. Printed instructions and explanations of any special preparation are desirable.
* *Ethics.* Operators should respect the privacy of patients and ensure the availability of adequate changing rooms, gowns, etc. Results of examinations should be released only as directed by the supervising physician. The use of ultrasound should be limited to recognized diagnostic and therapeutic purposes (determination of fetal sex, except as required for sex-linked disease screening, is not a medically valid reason for ultrasound examination).

- *Confidentiality.* The confidentiality of medical information (e.g. medical history and the results of sonographic examinations) should be respected.
- *Infection control.* Transducer cleaning and disinfection as necessary are essential for the control of infection. Established practice includes thorough cleaning with soap and water using a cleaning brush and immersion in cleaning solutions (e.g. chlorine, antiseptic). Other possible precautions should comply with established practice in the country.
- *Patient's rights.* The rights of the patient should always be respected, including the right to refuse to be examined; the patient's cultural and religious beliefs should be accorded consideration. The patient should be informed of any risks before examination, should be allowed to have a relative present if he or she wishes, and should be kept adequately informed during the course of the examination.
- *Medical equipment.* Sonographers and other allied health professionals who use diagnostic ultrasound should have an appropriate knowledge of medical equipment, including the operation of intravenous units, cardiac monitors, oxygen and suction equipment, catheters, chest and drainage pumps, and other equipment.
- *Patient's condition.* Sonographers should be able to assess the patient with respect to his or her level of consciousness and anxiety on the basis of respiration, colour, etc.
- *Medical terminology.* Sonographers should be familiar with the appropriate use of medical terminology.

4.4.7 *Principles of scanning*

Sonographers should be familiar with:

- generally accepted standards of image orientation;
- examination protocols;
- scanning planes;
- proper adjustment of equipment;
- the relation between frequency and resolution;
- scanning artefacts;
- permanent documentation of images.

4.4.8 *Requirements for teachers of sonographers*

Teachers should have successfully completed a course of at least the same level as that they teach. It is further suggested that teachers be accredited in their area of instruction. Appropriate accreditation could be granted by the national health authority, an academic institution, the national diagnostic ultrasound society, or another similar body. The Study Group recommends that teachers have at least a year of clinical experience in ultrasonography.

Teachers should regularly attend ultrasonography meetings and conferences to ensure that their knowledge of this rapidly developing field remains up to date. They should maintain an active and continuing involvement in clinical ultrasonography.

Section 6 further discusses the recommended requirements for teachers of ultrasonography.

4.4.9 *Evaluation*

Sonographers and other allied health professionals who use diagnostic ultrasound should, wherever possible, obtain recognition of their competence through established organizations granting recognized credentials. Countries without such an organization are encouraged to establish mechanisms to assess competence in ultrasonography. Examinations should assess knowledge of the material described above. It is further recommended that credentials be reassessed at regular intervals. Criteria based on competence in ultrasonography can be employed; whatever the criteria, the evaluation should be objective.

4.4.10 *Continuing medical education*

Continuing medical education is important for the maintenance of competence in ultrasonography. The Study Group recommends that sonographers and other allied health professionals using diagnostic ultrasound provide evidence of continuing medical education. Hospitals, medical schools, and government sponsored programmes should provide opportunities for such medical education.

4.4.11 *Specialized training*

Sonographers and other allied health professionals will need additional training to be able to use diagnostic ultrasound in specialized clinical areas requiring real-time, Doppler, duplex, and colour Doppler techniques. Such applications include cardiac, ophthalmic, and vascular ultrasonography.

Ultrasonography of the vascular system
Vascular technologists or allied health professionals performing ultrasound examinations of the vascular system should have an understanding of the anatomical structures, physiology, and haemodynamics of the vascular system. They should be able to recognize, identify, and appropriately document the sonographic appearance of

vascular disease. Other non-invasive techniques in addition to diagnostic ultrasound may be a required component of accreditation for the vascular use of diagnostic ultrasound.

Ultrasonography of the eye
An ophthalmic sonographer or allied health professional performing ultrasound examinations of the eye should be competent in the use and interpretation of real-time ultrasound. The use and interpretation of A-mode Doppler or colour Doppler ultrasound may also be required. The ophthalmic sonographer should be able to recognize and document the sonographic appearance of normal and abnormal intraocular and retrobulbar structures, as well as recognize, identify, and document ocular disease, foreign bodies, and trauma.

Ultrasonography of the heart
A cardiac sonographer or allied health professional performing ultrasound examinations of the heart should be able to recognize and identify the sonographic appearance of the anatomic structures of the heart and large vessels and to assess their physiology and haemodynamics by means of ultrasound. He or she should be able to recognize, identify, and appropriately document the sonographic appearance of acquired cardiac disease and congenital anomalies.

5. Basic sciences and instrumentation curricula

5.1 Introduction

An understanding of the basic physical and scientific principles underlying ultrasonography and its instrumentation is essential to achieve the maximum diagnostic benefit from this technology. A good foundation in basic principles will aid the user in obtaining diagnostic information with the ultrasound scanner while avoiding common pitfalls that impair diagnosis.

The curriculum in basic sciences and instrumentation has two main objectives:

- to provide the ultrasonography practitioner with sufficient knowledge to operate the ultrasound scanner effectively and obtain the necessary data, with due regard for data quality and patient safety;
- to provide an understanding of the nature of the artefacts that may be present in ultrasonographic data, so that they can be recognized and errors in interpretation can be avoided.

The curriculum has two parts. The first is intended for those who will practise general ultrasonography (physicians and non-physicians, mainly with a general purpose ultrasound scanner) and should be taught to all those following one of the level I ultrasonography curricula. The second part contains additional information required for those following an advanced or specialized curriculum using more sophisticated equipment (*32*). Completion of the first part is a prerequisite for undertaking the second part. The two, however, can be combined into a single course covering all material.

5.2 Prerequisites

The curriculum assumes knowledge of mathematics and physics sufficient to understand the material presented.

5.2.1 *Mathematics*

A basic knowledge of mathematics is required to understand the concepts of ultrasound. The following list of topics is representative:

- graphs (concepts necessary for understanding ultrasound displays);
- algebra (i.e. manipulation of a simple equation);
- trigonometry (for understanding the Doppler equation);
- logarithms (for decibel (dB) notation).

Note: The latter two topics are necessary only for the advanced curriculum.

5.2.2 *Physics*

Knowledge of the following physical quantities and principles is necessary for adequate comprehension of the basics of ultrasonography:

- frequency;
- force and pressure;
- density;
- speed and velocity;
- simple wave motion;
- basic electricity.

5.2.3 *Biology*

Some knowledge of biology is necessary to understand the tissue reflection and scattering of ultrasound waves, and for an appreciation of the possible biological effects and safe use of ultrasound:

- blood and blood flow (tissue perfusion and cooling);
- cells and organs (the cell cycle and cellular susceptibility to damage);

- tissue types (according to ultrasound transmission and reflection properties like average wave speed, attenuation, and echogenicity):
  — soft (i.e. average speed and attenuation);
  — hard (e.g. bone);
  — cystic (e.g. polycystic kidney);
  — solid (e.g. muscle, liver);
  — calcified (e.g. certain diseased cardiac valves, atheromatous plaques);
  — complex (e.g. malignant tumour, placenta);
  — gas containing (e.g. lung, alimentary tract).

5.3 Basic sciences and instrumentation curriculum for general ultrasonography

5.3.1 *Basic sciences*

Physics

The concepts necessary for understanding the properties of ultrasound as used for clinical examination include:

- the definition of ultrasound;
- frequency, sound speed, and wavelength;
- reflection (at perpendicular and oblique incidence) and scattering;
- wave attenuation;
- dB notation;
- useful frequency ranges;
- generation and detection of ultrasound waves;
- pulse–echo principle and the range equation;
- the Doppler phenomenon (basics only).

Biological effects and safety

The operator will need to be familiar with the circumstances in which caution in instrument settings should be exercised so that the recommended maximum exposure limits are not approached:

- the safety record of clinical use (see p. 2);
- the safety guidelines that should be observed:
  — mechanical and thermal safety indices (it is important to cover the phenomenon of cavitation);
  — maximum energy output (varies according to machine);
- non-ultrasonic safety aspects:
  — contamination;
  — electric shock;
  — thermal injury (from excessive probe temperature);
  — mechanical injury (e.g. from improper use of endoprobes).

Imaging methods

To understand the scanning protocols used for particular examinations and the artefacts that can be produced, the operator will require knowledge of the following elements of image formation:

- the pulse–echo principles of image generation (range equation);
- the principles of ultrasound beam formation and focusing (both spatial and temporal resolution);
- the ultrasound display modes commonly used:
  — two-dimensional mode;
  — M-mode (fundamentals only);
- ultrasound beam steering and corresponding scan formats (rectilinear, sector, parallelogram);
- the relation of frame rate and real-time scanning;
- the principles of grey-scale imaging:
  — dynamic range (in dB) and possibilities for image post-processing;
  — tissue echogenicity (i.e. "texture" as represented in grey-scale);
  — artefacts that can enhance diagnostic accuracy (e.g. shadows).

5.3.2 *Equipment*

The operator should be familiar with the following aspects of ultrasound equipment:

- operating frequency (choice varies depending on average wave penetration, attenuation, scattering, etc.);
- scan format and probe type (choice depends on the size of the scanned anatomical plane and the possibility of access via acoustic "windows");
- scanner controls:
  — ultrasound power output;
  — overall receiver gain, swept gain (e.g. time gain compensation);
  — focal length;
- display controls:
  — brightness;
  — contrast;
  — image selection and storage (freeze-frame);
- image-record features:
  — patient identification;
  — indication of distance scale (use of calipers);
  — calculations of gestational age from biparietal diameter, cross-sectional areas, etc.;
- image-recording capabilities (e.g. self-processing or not, single or multiformat):

— film;
— video printer;
— video cassette recorder.

5.3.3 *Quality assurance*

Although ultrasound scanners of the recent generation are much more stable than older ones, it is important to implement a programme of quality assurance to ensure that a deterioration in equipment performance does not affect the quality of diagnosis (*33*). The specific features of the quality-assurance programme should be determined with regard to local circumstances. As a minimum, scans of a standard object obtained with standard machine settings should be recorded and retained on file. A standard object can be either a fixed element of the operator's anatomy, when appropriate, such as the mesenteric artery, or a "phantom". Phantoms simulate human tissue and blood flow properties and can be scanned for quality-assurance purposes. Past scans should be reviewed after each regular quality-assurance check, in order to detect any deterioration in image quality.

The following aspects of image quality should be checked routinely:

- spatial resolution (i.e. the ability to separate closely spaced reflectors);
- contrast resolution (i.e. the ability to distinguish between small differences in echogenicity).

5.3.4 *Equipment management*

The ultrasound operator should be able to make appropriate decisions about the following aspects of equipment management:

- the specifications to request when purchasing (e.g. appropriateness for intended use, compatibility with local power supply, etc.);
- acceptance testing (does the machine match the initial specifications?);
- machine maintenance and repair (the operator will need to take into account the availability of spare parts and the possibility of arranging for support by service technicians);
- equipment life-cycle (including plans for machine replacement and long-term cost estimates).

5.3.5 *Artefacts*

The ability to recognize the wide variety of artefacts that occur in ultrasonic images is vital for correct diagnostic interpretation. This recognition requires a good knowledge of the topics already mentioned, as well as of the following specific subjects.

The operator should thoroughly understand the basic assumptions of good image formation:

- propagation of straight, narrow ultrasound beams for geometrical accuracy;
- avoidance of multiple pulse reflection;
- use of a constant sound-speed for accurate image registration and distance measurement.

The operator should also be familiar with the following common artefacts:

- beam-width artefacts, affected by:
  — beam width;
  — beam sidelobes;
  — beam (slice) thickness;
- multiple reflection artefacts:
  — mirror reflection;
  — reverberation;
- acoustic shadowing, enhancement, and attenuation;
- refraction artefacts:
  — geometrical distortion or duplication;
  — changes in image intensity.

5.4 Basic sciences and instrumentation curriculum for advanced ultrasonography

The following curriculum is designed for more advanced applications of ultrasound and should be taught together with the clinical curriculum described in section 3.3. The actual topics covered should be appropriate to the techniques used in the particular ultrasound practice. It is assumed that all the material in the basic sciences and instrumentation curriculum for general ultrasound has been mastered before the following material is presented.

5.4.1 *Basic sciences*

It is expected that at the successful completion of this curriculum the graduate will have an understanding that is both broader and deeper than that of a graduate of a general (level I) ultrasonography course, normally oriented towards use of a general purpose ultrasound scanner.

Physics
Ultrasonography practice with the sophisticated equipment available at levels II and III requires an understanding of the following:

- units of intensity used for acoustic output specification;

* advanced-level theory of the Doppler effect;
* the use of contrast agents (e.g. encapsulated gas microbubbles).

Biological effects and safety

This section should provide an understanding of the phenomena involved in potential effects of ultrasound on biological tissue, rather than a simple description of required safety limits.

Biological tissues can be affected by:

* thermal mechanisms (can cause, for example, the coagulation of proteins);
* non-thermal mechanisms (e.g. destruction of cell membranes due to streaming);
* the use of Doppler techniques (sometimes involving higher power output than non-Doppler ultrasound);
* the use of contrast agents (may enhance cavitation);
* the use of endoprobes (risk of physical injury);
* interventional techniques (risk of infection).

Imaging methods

The advanced course should include a more detailed study of equipment capabilities and the factors affecting equipment performance. The following topics should be covered:

* beam focal zones during the pulse (transmit) and echo (receive) phase;
* frame rate according to pulse rate and image complexity;
* making measurements from M-mode recording;
* dynamic range;
* factors affecting needle visualization, particularly the tip, during ultrasonically guided puncture.

Doppler methods

As only basic Doppler theory is covered in the general ultrasound curriculum, the presentation for the advanced course should start at an elementary level, including:

* continuous wave and pulsed mode Doppler ultrasound;
* operating frequency (determined by the wave-scattering properties of, for example, blood, and the wave attenuation of overlying tissue);
* frequency spectral display (visualization of the energy and time distribution of Doppler frequencies);
* control of aliasing (occurs when the pulse repetition frequency is less than twice the highest Doppler shift frequency);

- Doppler analysis:
  — determination of true velocity from the Doppler frequency and the angle between the scanning beam and the measured velocity;
  — determination of the frequency spectrum (for derivation of the Doppler shift frequency and for indication of flow disturbance).

Combined methods

Both duplex scanning (two-dimensional real-time imaging containing a single line of Doppler information) and colour Doppler scanning use a combination of Doppler and non-Doppler techniques. The following elements should be covered:

- velocity determination and frequency spectral display (duplex scanning);
- frequency, power, velocity, and selection of colour scale (colour Doppler).

5.4.2 Equipment

Real-time scanner

The following features are present in sophisticated machines but not in a general purpose ultrasound scanner:

- focal-zone selection;
- frame-rate selection;
- intracavitary probes.

Continuous-wave Doppler

The continuous-wave Doppler technique is used mainly in ultrasound studies of the vascular system and in fetal heart monitoring. It typically offers:

- audio output of the Doppler shift frequency;
- display of heart rate as measured by Doppler ultrasound;
- frequency spectral display;
- Doppler filters for elimination of irrelevant signals;
- paper chart recording.

Pulsed-wave Doppler

Pulsed-wave Doppler is used when discrimination in distance to the target or region giving rise to Doppler signals is required. It involves:

- selection of sample window (depth and length);
- selection of pulse repetition frequency.

Colour flow imaging
Certain features are specific to colour flow imaging:

- colour scale selection (colour is used to represent flow velocity and flow direction; usually red indicates flow towards the probe, and blue, flow away from the probe);
- the write-priority setting (can suppress the display of colour when the echogenicity exceeds a chosen threshold, which helps to distinguish solid tissue);
- size selection of colour display region (usually kept as small as possible to allow higher frame rate);
- beam steering (particularly with linear array scanners);
- spectral variance display (indicating flow disturbance and usually displayed in green).

Power imaging
Power imaging displays the amount of blood flow (as measured by Doppler power) within a grey-scale image of surrounding tissue. The operator should be familiar with the proper adjustment of:

- colour gain (determines the minimum quantity of flow necessary to produce a colour display);
- frequency threshold (sets the minimum flow velocity necessary for colour display);
- intensity threshold (suppresses echoes from solid tissue).

5.4.3 *Quality assurance*

Quality assurance for advanced operators should cover:

- a review of material related to quality assurance from the general ultrasound curriculum;
- the use of Doppler phantoms (containing moving targets or a liquid simulating blood flow);
- correct use and disinfection of endoprobes.

5.4.4 *Artefacts*

Doppler techniques are associated with a number of specific artefacts. The advanced ultrasound operator will need to be able to recognize these as well as acquire a deeper understanding of, and better ability to recognize, the artefacts discussed in the general ultrasound course. The trainee should become familiar with:

- multiple reflection artefacts with Doppler ultrasound:
  — mirror reflection;
  — reverberation;

- two kinds of Doppler aliasing:
  — frequency spectral aliasing (occurs when the Doppler shift frequency exceeds half the pulse repetition frequency);
  — range ambiguity (occurs when pulse repetition frequency exceeds the reciprocal of echo time);
- artefacts due to colour frame rate that can occur when the frame rate is so slow that changes occur in flow conditions during frame acquisition.

5.5 Course duration

Each basic science and instrumentation course (general and advanced) should require 20 hours of instruction time.

5.6 Evaluation

A practical evaluation of the trainee's ability to operate the scanner and correctly interpret scans is the most important measure of achievement with respect to the curriculum. A written examination is also important.

6. Training centres and resources

High-quality, cost-effective training for physicians and allied health professionals performing diagnostic ultrasound procedures is needed worldwide. The rapid dissemination of ultrasound equipment of all levels of sophistication, with very often no local restrictions on purchase or utilization, exacerbates the need for such education.

6.1 Needs and priorities

Training needs in developed and developing countries are different. While both need adequately trained personnel, the ability to provide them varies significantly (see section 1.1). In many developed countries, national diagnostic ultrasound societies and governmental organizations have together developed standards or recommendations for training and, in some countries, accreditation. In these countries, awareness of the need for high standards of practice in ultrasonography has in some cases led to the official recognition of training institutions as well as accreditation of individual practitioners. However, even in developed countries, there is concern about the improper or inappropriate use of diagnostic ultrasound and about the acquisition and use of ultrasonography equipment by those who are not properly trained to use it. In developing countries, the scarcity of appropriately educated physicians has led to a much greater potential for users of diagnostic ultrasound to have insufficient training, increasing the possibilities of inappropriate diagnoses and incomplete or incorrect treatment. Moreover, governmental controls and organizational guidelines are more often lacking in developing countries.

This report has established some principles for adequate training in diagnostic ultrasound at both basic and advanced levels. In addition, the need for the proper organization of training programmes and of support for teachers and infrastructure, including educational centres and teaching materials, has been indicated.

6.2 Teacher training

The training of ultrasonography teachers is a fundamental element of any strategy to implement this report's recommendations. Effective teaching requires not only a thorough knowledge of the subject matter, but also a high level of interest in teaching and the willingness to devote time and effort to achieve excellence. To be an effective ultrasonography teacher, an individual must have a thorough understanding of all aspects of the use of diagnostic ultrasound and must have attained professional competence at a level no less than that required of his or her students. Ideally, the teacher's knowledge should be greater than that required of his or her students. An example of the ideal teacher in ultrasonography is an experienced sonologist or sonographer actively performing clinical ultrasound examinations in the specialty areas in which he or she is teaching. However, courses in basic science and instrumentation may be provided by a scientist or engineer with the appropriate background in ultrasonography. Experience in all aspects of general ultrasonography for teaching at the basic level is required; more advanced training needs teachers with either higher levels of competence in general ultrasonography or expertise in particular areas of specialization. In addition to a thorough knowledge of ultrasonography and clinical expertise, teachers should also have a good understanding of techniques and methodologies of pedagogy. Although this can be obtained from specialized teacher-training programmes, it is also recognized that such expertise can be obtained from years of experience in teaching ultrasonography. Thus, a specialized certificate in teaching, although not a necessity, has been recognized as helpful in some countries.

Recommendations of state, regional, or national organizations should be taken into account by ultrasonography instructors in formulating their course plans and in their actual teaching. This report provides an outline of the information that should be covered in training programmes at various levels; however, modifications should be made according to regional variations in the prevalence of disease, or other factors (*34*).

6.3 Material and techniques

Ultrasonography teachers should endeavour to make use of all available training materials and technologies. Wherever possible, conventional didactic lectures should be supplemented by directed reading in textbooks, published procedure protocols, and journal articles. In addition, videotape, CD-ROM, and interactive media are valuable means of extending the coverage of material taught. Interactive diagnostic ultrasound simulators will probably become available in the future and should prove useful for increasing skills (*35, 36*). Instruction in scanning techniques and extensive hands-on experience under supervision is also an important aspect of training. Obtaining sufficient hands-on experience with patients may require the student to undergo a training period away from the primary didactic learning site, as the availability of specific types of clinical experience may vary from site to site. Outside expertise should also be used whenever possible: in ideal circumstances, training would be provided not only by individuals permanently associated with the training centre but also by invited lecturers who can provide a different perspective. However, cost plays an important role, and a reasonable substitute would be the use of videotapes and CD-ROMs from a variety of sources. In the future, satellite and other communication links may open new possibilities for distance learning. Electronic teaching aids are becoming increasingly available worldwide and can provide a valuable supplement to a training programme provided they are used with the guidance of an on-site teacher.

6.4 Evaluation

Where appropriate, the use of both pre-training and post-training examinations is recommended (i.e. written and practical examinations). Whenever possible, examinations should be developed by experts other than the teaching staff so that the performance of both teachers and students can be impartially evaluated. Such examinations should not preclude or substitute for those prepared by the teacher to provide regular feedback concerning the effectiveness of teaching and students' capabilities for assimilating and utilizing knowledge provided in the training programme.

6.5 Teacher-training programmes

The development and implementation of intensive training programmes specifically for ultrasonography instructors is desirable and has been established practice for many years in some countries (e.g. Germany). Models of such programmes have been developed at the Jefferson Ultrasound Research and Education Institute in the United States, at present the only recognized WHO Collaborating Centre for Continuing and General Education in Diagnostic Ultrasound. In the Jefferson Institute programmes, participants receive not only the latest information about clinical and technical knowledge in the field in which they are going to teach, but also instruction in the methods and techniques of teaching. Programmes such as these should be developed at other major training centres throughout the world.

6.6 Licensing and accreditation

Licensing and accreditation of ultrasound practitioners and teachers are the responsibility of local, national, or regional governmental authorities, professional societies, or other recognized organizations. Licensing and accreditation programmes vary widely from country to country (see section 2). In general, a formal system of accreditation helps raise the standard of ultrasonography practice.

6.7 Continuing education

Regardless of the level of expertise acquired, all instructors and practitioners of ultrasonography should pursue continuing education through "refresher" courses and conferences, as well as those offering updates on new technology and practice. The latter are particularly important if the individual wishes to expand his or her expertise into new areas. Periodic reaccreditation is also highly desirable.

6.8 Training centres

Particularly in countries where there is the greatest need for qualified practitioners and instructors, it is advisable that regional and national training centres be established, either independently or associated with an established educational institution, (e.g. a university or university hospital).

6.8.1 *Regional (international) centres*

Regional centres should be established with the collaboration of all countries in a region, and preferably with the assistance of international professional organizations.

The principal responsibilities of a regional centre should include:

- the collection and dissemination of information on all aspects of ultrasonography, including new techniques and developments in equipment;
- the development of training programmes for those who will use diagnostic ultrasound in patient care;
- the training of instructors of ultrasonography;
- the maintenance of the quality of teaching in national training centres within the region;
- the establishment and maintenance of standards for qualifying examinations (in some regions, examinations may be the responsibility of the regional centre and should in such cases be recognized and accepted in each country in the region).

6.8.2 *National centres*

National centres should be recognized by relevant national authorities and professional organizations and should have the right to hold examinations and issue diplomas or certificates after satisfactory completion of a recognized course of study. It is highly desirable that well qualified experts from other institutions and professional societies be involved in the assessment process.

National centres should maintain practice equipment and a library of print and audiovisual material.

National centres should ensure that locally important diseases receive proper attention.

Both regional and national centres can be important for improving the standard of ultrasonography. Both should be involved in and promote research on local health problems and provide information to other countries.

6.9 Equipment

Training centres should have adequate equipment and should be responsible for the implementation of educational programmes.

6.9.1 *Ultrasound equipment*

For level I training, a general purpose ultrasound scanner is required.

For more advanced training, the equipment and transducers appropriate to the subjects taught are required. This equipment should be of the current generation and should have been distributed within the region within the last 3–5 years.

Equipment for image recording should be available and used routinely during training. Such equipment should include videotape-recording, a hard-copy device, and image storage facilities.

Equipment for training should be well maintained and subject to regular quality assurance checks. As far as possible, training equipment should be of the same type that will be used after qualification.

6.9.2 *Training equipment*

The use of tissue-simulating phantoms is desirable for testing spatial and contrast resolutions. Phantoms or dummies for practising scanning and ultrasonically guided puncture (where appropriate) are also desirable.

Videotape and 35-mm slide-viewing facilities should be provided.

6.10 **Access to patients**

Training centres should have access to patients presenting a range of conditions appropriate for the areas taught.

6.11 **Space and equipment requirements**

The space available for scanning and instruction should be consistent with the number of trainees to be accommodated. One scanner for each five trainees is desirable, but no more than ten trainees should be assigned to a single scanner. Appropriate classroom and study space should be available for all students.

7. **Conclusions and recommendations**

1. The appropriate training of the users of diagnostic ultrasound is the most important requisite for the improvement and rational application of ultrasonography in medical practice. The use of diagnostic ultrasound by individuals with inadequate knowledge and skills increases the likelihood of unnecessary patient examinations and misdiagnosis and imposes additional costs on the health care system.
2. The purchase and use of diagnostic ultrasound equipment should be restricted to those who have successfully completed an adequate training programme or have achieved a proven level of competence in ultrasonography. The Study Group endorses the conclusion of the WHO Scientific Group on the Future Use of New Imaging Technologies in Developing Countries that the "purchase of ultrasound equipment without making provision for the training of an operator is contrary to good health care practice and is unlikely to be cost-effective" (9).
3. The Study Group strongly recommends that appropriate curricula should be adopted for the general, advanced, and specialized train-

ing of medical doctors and allied health professionals who use diagnostic ultrasound. Examples of such curricula have been provided (see sections 3–5).

4. WHO, international governmental and nongovernmental organizations, and professional associations should be actively involved in the development of training programmes for the use of diagnostic ultrasound. Such involvement should include setting training standards and organizing and carrying out training courses (with accreditation of trainees) together with continuing education programmes.

5. Since diagnostic ultrasound technology is developing rapidly, regular equipment upgrading is essential, particularly in institutions where training is provided.

6. The equipment, training, and practice of ultrasonography should be oriented towards local health care problems, and should have a positive effect on the quality of health care in the country concerned.

Acknowledgements

The Study Group wishes to thank the World Federation for Ultrasound in Medicine and Biology for its financial support and active participation in the preparation of the meeting. The Study Group would also like to thank the WHO Collaborating Centre for Continuing and General Education in Diagnostic Ultrasound (Jefferson Ultrasound Research and Education Institute) as well as the Thomas Jefferson University, in particular its President P.C. Brucker and Vice-President J.J. Saukkonen, for making available secretarial and other administrative support and for graciously hosting the meeting. The helpful assistance of Dr C. Borras, Regional Adviser, WHO Regional Office for the Americas, was also appreciated.

References

1. Goldberg BB, Kimmelman BA. *Medical diagnostic ultrasound: a retrospective on its 40th anniversary.* Rochester, NY, Eastman Kodak, 1988:1–49.

2. Wells PNJ. The prudent use of diagnostic ultrasound. *Ultrasound in medicine and biology*, 1987, **13**:391–400.

3. Bioeffects considerations for the safety of diagnostic ultrasound. American Institute of Ultrasound in Medicine. Bioeffects Committee. *Journal of ultrasound in medicine*, 1988, **7**(Suppl. 9).

4. WFUMB Symposium on Safety and Standardisation in Medical Ultrasound. Issues and recommendations regarding thermal mechanisms for biological effects of ultrasound. Hornbaek, Denmark, 30 August–1 September 1991. *Ultrasound in medicine and biology*, 1992, **18**:731–810.

5. *Bioeffects and safety of diagnostic ultrasound.* Laurel, MD, American Institute of Ultrasound in Medicine, 1993.

6. *Medical ultrasound safety. Part I: Bioeffects and biophysics. Part II: Prudent use. Part III: Implementing ALARA.* Laurel, MD, American Institute of Ultrasound in Medicine, 1994.

7. **Larsen JF, Larsen T.** Unskilled ultrasound scanning in gynecology and obstetrics can lead to serious risks [in Danish]. *Ugeskrift for Læger*, 1991, **153**:2187–2188.

8. **Bundy AL.** Legal concerns in diagnostic ultrasound: an overview. In: Fleischer AC et al, eds. *Sonography in obstetrics and gynecology: principles and practice.* 5th ed. Stamford, CT, Appleton & Lange, 1996:1027–1031.

9. *Future use of new imaging technologies in developing countries. Report of a WHO Scientific Group.* Geneva, World Health Organization, 1985 (WHO Technical Report Series, No. 723).

10. *Effective choices for diagnostic imaging in clinical practice. Report of a WHO Scientific Group.* Geneva, World Health Organization, 1990 (WHO Technical Report Series, No. 795).

11. **Palmer PES, ed.** *Manual of diagnostic ultrasound.* Geneva, World Health Organization, 1995.

12. *The control of schistosomiasis. Second report of the WHO Expert Committee.* Geneva, World Health Organization, 1993 (WHO Technical Report Series, No. 830).

13. **Kurjak A, Breyer B.** The use of ultrasound in developing countries. *Ultrasound in medicine and biology*, 1986, **12**:611–621.

14. *Rational use of diagnostic imaging in paediatrics. Report of a WHO Study Group.* Geneva, World Health Organization, 1987 (WHO Technical Report Series, No. 757).

15. *Syllabus and regulations for the certificate examination in medical ultrasound and the award of the diploma in medical ultrasound.* London, College of Radiographers, 1988.

16. **Sjöberg N-O, Maršàl K.** Postgraduate education in ultrasound diagnosis in obstetrics and gynaecology in Sweden. *Early human development*, 1992, **29**:117–120.

17. *Basic ultrasound training for general practitioners. Report of a Joint Working Party.* London, Royal College of General Practitioners & Royal College of Radiologists, 1993.

18. *Educational guidelines for diagnostic sonography.* Rockville, MD, American Institute of Ultrasound in Medicine, 1993.

19. *Diploma of medical ultrasonography: handbook.* Willoughby, New South Wales, Australasian Society for Ultrasound in Medicine, 1995.

20. **Filly RA.** Radiology residency training in diagnostic sonography: recommendations of the Society of Radiologists in Ultrasound. *Radiology*, 1989, **172**:577.

21. **Smith CB et al.** Quantification of training in obstetrical ultrasound: a study of family practice residents. *Journal of clinical ultrasound*, 1991, **19**:479–483.

22. **Ahram J, Feinstein SJ, De Phillips H.** Survey of ultrasound training in obstetrics and gynecology residency training programs in the United States. *Obstetrics and gynecology*, 1987, **70**:405–407.

23. **Moreau JF, Bessis R, Le Guern H**. L'ultrasonographie médicale en France: propositions pour le futur. [Medical ultrasonography in France: proposals for the future.] *Journal d'échographie et de médecine ultrasonore*, 1991, **12**:258–263.

24. Sonderdruck aus Verträgen der kassenärztlichen Bundesvereinigung. Ultraschallvereinbarung vom 10 Februar 1993. [Reprint of the contracts of the Federal Health Insurance Association. Ultrasound agreement of 10 February 1993.] Germany, Federal Health Insurance Association, 1993.

25. *Essentials and guidelines of an accredited educational program for the diagnostic medical sonographer.* USA, Joint Review Committee on Education in Diagnostic Medical Sonography, 1987.

26. *The scope of practice for the diagnostic sonographer.* Dallas, TX, Society of Diagnostic Medical Sonographers, 1993.

27. *Examination information & application.* Cincinnati, OH, American Registry of Diagnostic Medical Sonographers, 1995 (unpublished document available on request from American Registry of Diagnostic Medical Sonographers, 2368 Victory Parkway, Suite 510, Cincinnati, OH, 45206).

28. *International survey on radiation medicine technology.* Tokyo, Japanese Association of Radiological Technologists, 1995.

29. *Guidelines for obstetrics and gynecology review.* Dallas, TX, Society of Diagnostic Medical Sonographers, 1992.

30. *Guidelines for abdomen review.* Dallas, TX, Society of Diagnostic Medical Sonographers, 1994.

31. The role of the sonographer (February 1996). *Australasian Society for Ultrasound in Medicine newsletter*, April 1996:13–14.

32. *Standard for real-time display of thermal and mechanical acoustic output indices on diagnostic ultrasound equipment.* Rockville, MD and Washington, DC, American Institute of Ultrasound in Medicine and National Electrical Manufacturers Association, 1992.

33. *AIUM quality assurance manual for gray-scale ultrasound scanners. Stage 2.* Laurel, MD, American Institute of Ultrasound in Medicine, 1995.

34. *Increasing the relevance of education for health professionals. Report of a WHO Study Group on Problem-Solving Education for the Health Professions.* Geneva, World Health Organization, 1993 (WHO Technical Report Series, No. 838).

35. **Ville Y et al.** Development of training model for ultrasound-guided invasive procedures in fetal medicine. *Ultrasound in obstetrics and gynecology*, 1995, **5**:180–183.

36. **Lee W et al.** Interactive multimedia for prenatal ultrasound training. *Obstetrics and gynaecology*, 1995, **85**:135–140.

Selected further reading

The Study Group noted that a number of documents related to the maintenance of high standards of practice in ultrasonography are already being distributed by various organizations.

American Institute of Ultrasound in Medicine

1. *Ultrasound practice accreditation: standards and guidelines for the accreditation of ultrasound practices.* 1996.
2. *Guidelines for performance of the abdominal and retroperitoneal ultrasound examination.* 1994.
3. *Guidelines for performance of the ultrasound examination of the female pelvis.* 1995.
4. *Guidelines for performance of the ultrasound examination of the prostate and surrounding structures.* 1991.

(Available on request from American Institute of Ultrasound in Medicine, 14750 Sweitzer Lane, Suite 100, Laurel, MD 20707-5906, USA.)

Australasian Society for Ultrasound in Medicine

5. *Guidelines for the 18–20 week obstetrical scan.* 1991.
6. *Guidelines for the performance of third trimester ultrasound.* 1995.
7. *Policy on ultrasonographer training.* 1988.

(Available on request from Australasian Society for Ultrasound in Medicine, 2/181 High Street, Willoughby, New South Wales, 2065, Australia.)

World Health Organization

8. *Meeting on ultrasonography in schistosomiasis. Proposal for a practical guide to the standardized use of ultrasound in the assessment of pathological changes, 1–4 October 1990, Cairo, Egypt.* Geneva, World Health Organization, 1991, Annex A (unpublished document TDR/SCH/ULTRASON/91.3, available on request from Special Programme for Research and Training in Tropical Diseases, World Health Organization, 1211 Geneva 27, Switzerland).

Annex
Applications of diagnostic ultrasound

Diagnostic ultrasound is used in nearly all fields of medicine and is the primary imaging modality in a large number of clinical situations. It is also widely employed as a secondary imaging modality for a broad range of conditions. Diagnostic ultrasound is an integral part of the practice of radiology, cardiology, internal medicine, surgery, and obstetrics. Its high clinical usefulness coupled with the relatively low-cost equipment and lack of ionizing radiation are resulting in its incorporation into a growing number of clinical specialties for both general and specialized applications. Examples of the common uses of diagnostic ultrasound grouped by specialty are shown in the following table. Some variation in applications occurs from country to country.

Specialty	Applications
Radiology	All paediatric examinations
	Neck, thyroid, and parathyroid
	Chest and mediastinum
	Heart
	Breast
	Abdominal organs, peritoneum, and retroperitoneum
	Female pelvis
	Scrotal contents
	Obstetric examinations
	Soft tissues, bone, muscles, tendons, and joints
	Visceral arteries and veins
	Peripheral arteries and veins
	Intraoperative applications
	Interventional procedures (biopsy, aspiration, etc.)
Cardiology	Heart
	Large vessels
Obstetrics	Fetus
	Uterus
	Placenta
Gynaecology	Uterus
	Ovaries
	Adnexa
Neurology and neurosurgery	Extracranial arteries
	Intracranial arteries
	Brain
Paediatrics	Brain
	Hips
	Abdomen

	Pelvis
	Heart
	Soft tissues
	Scrotal contents
Gastroenterology	Gastrointestinal tract
	Liver
	Biliary system
	Pancreas
	Spleen
Urology	Adrenals
	Kidneys
	Ureters
	Urinary bladder
	Prostate
	Seminal vesicles
	Scrotal contents
Surgery (including general, orthopaedic, vascular, and gastroenterological surgery)	Abdomen (for trauma)
	Intraoperative examinations (brain, spine, colon, and rectum)
	Pelvis
	Interventional procedures (biopsy, aspiration, etc.)
	Breast
	Soft tissues
	Joints and bones
	Extracranial arteries and veins
	Large vessels
Angiology	Peripheral arteries and veins
	Extracranial arteries
Internal medicine	Abdominal organs
	Retroperitoneal organs
	Chest and mediastinum
	Other parts (excluding breast, scrotum)
	Visceral and peripheral arteries and veins
	Heart (as a subspecialty)
	Infectious diseases (e.g. schistosomiasis and echinococcosis)